THE ULTIMATE ANTI-INFLAMMATORY DIET COOKBOOKFOR SENIORS

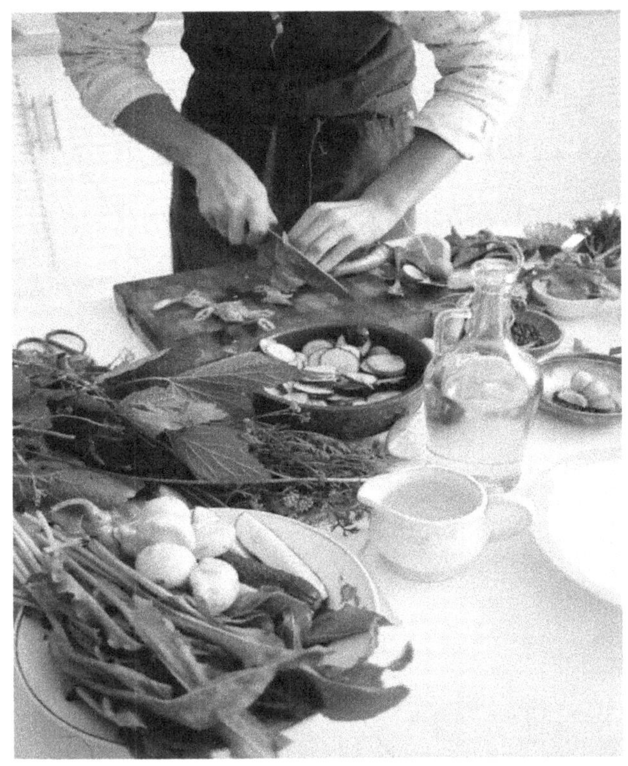

Quick and Easy Recipes to Detox Your Body, Relieve Your Persistent Pains and Restore Your Health

Mary D. Johnson

The Ultimate Anti-inflammatory Diet Cookbook for Seniors

Copyright © 2024 [Mary D. Johnson]

All rights reserved. No part of this publication may be reproduced, distributed, or transmitted in any form or by any means, including photocopying, recording, or other electronic or mechanical methods, without the prior written permission of the publisher, except in the case of brief quotations embodied in critical reviews and certain other noncommercial uses permitted by copyright law. For permission requests, write to the publisher at the address below:

[mary.d.johnson@gmail.com]

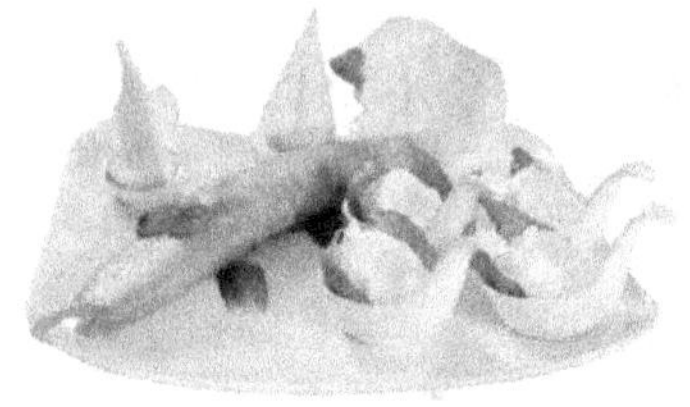

TABLE OF CONTENTS

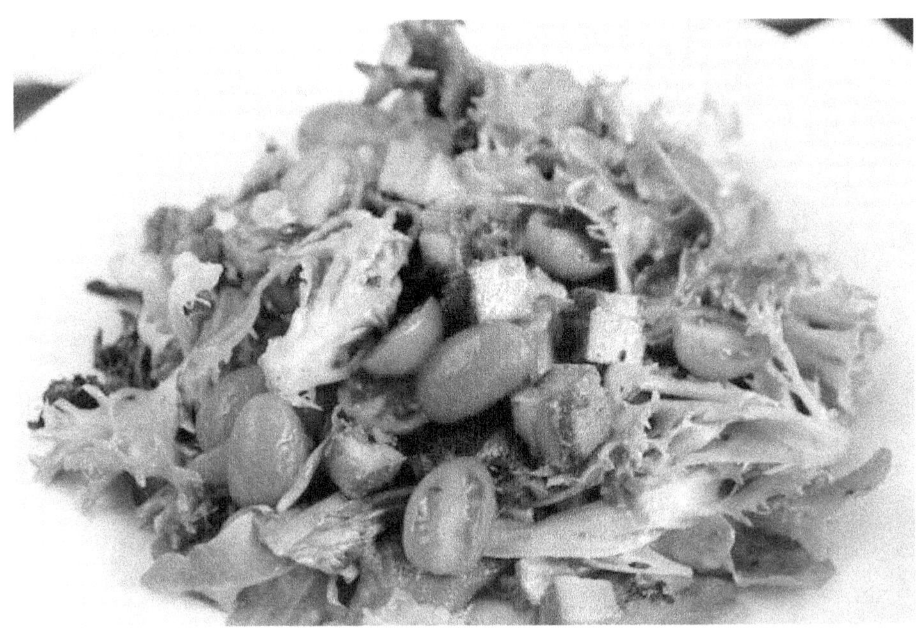

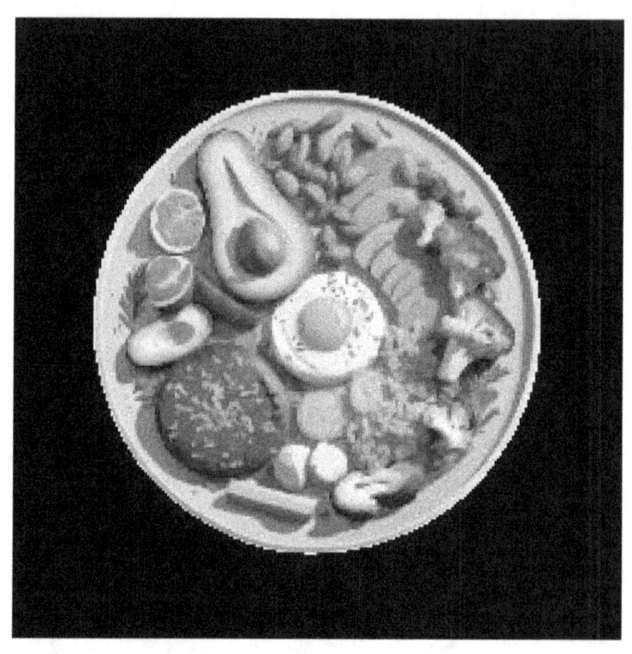

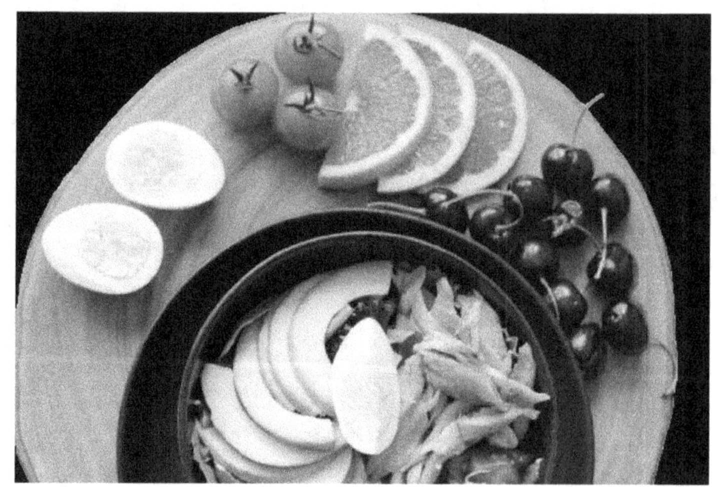

INTRODUCTION

When I was growing up, one of my father's business associates, Mr. Dickson, a vibrant middle-aged man then, used to come around our home to see my father and they often went out together to play golf. They equally used to spend time together over most weekends walking in the park, enjoying the fresh air and the beauty of nature. They really felt connected to the world and were full of life.

However, as the years passed, Dickson began to suffer from various inflammatory diseases. His joints ached, his energy waned, and the simple pleasure of walking became a painful ordeal. The inflammation in his body left him bedridden and despondent. He suffered in this condition for several years without lasting solution.

Last Christmas, my father visited his friend, Mr. Dickson, and gave him a thoughtful gift: a copy of my book, *Anti-inflammatory Diet Cookbook for Seniors*. Intrigued and with nothing to lose, Dickson decided to read the book. He found it to be a beacon of hope, filled with easy-to-follow recipes and nutritional advice specifically tailored to combat inflammation.

Determined to reclaim his health, Dickson began to implement the recommendations from the book. He swapped out processed foods for fresh vegetables, fruits, and whole grains. He started incorporating anti-inflammatory ingredients like turmeric, ginger, and omega-3-rich fish into his diet. Day by day, meal by meal, he followed the recipes and advice with unwavering dedication.

Gradually, Dickson noticed changes. His pain lessened, his energy levels increased, and his mood brightened. The inflammation in his body began to subside, and he started to regain his strength. Encouraged by his progress, Dickson continued on this new dietary path, finding joy in cooking and eating nourishing meals.

Months passed, and the transformation was remarkable. Dickson was no longer bedridden. He returned to his beloved park walks, greeting each day with renewed vigor and enthusiasm. The diet had given him a new lease on life, allowing him to enjoy his old vibrant self once more.

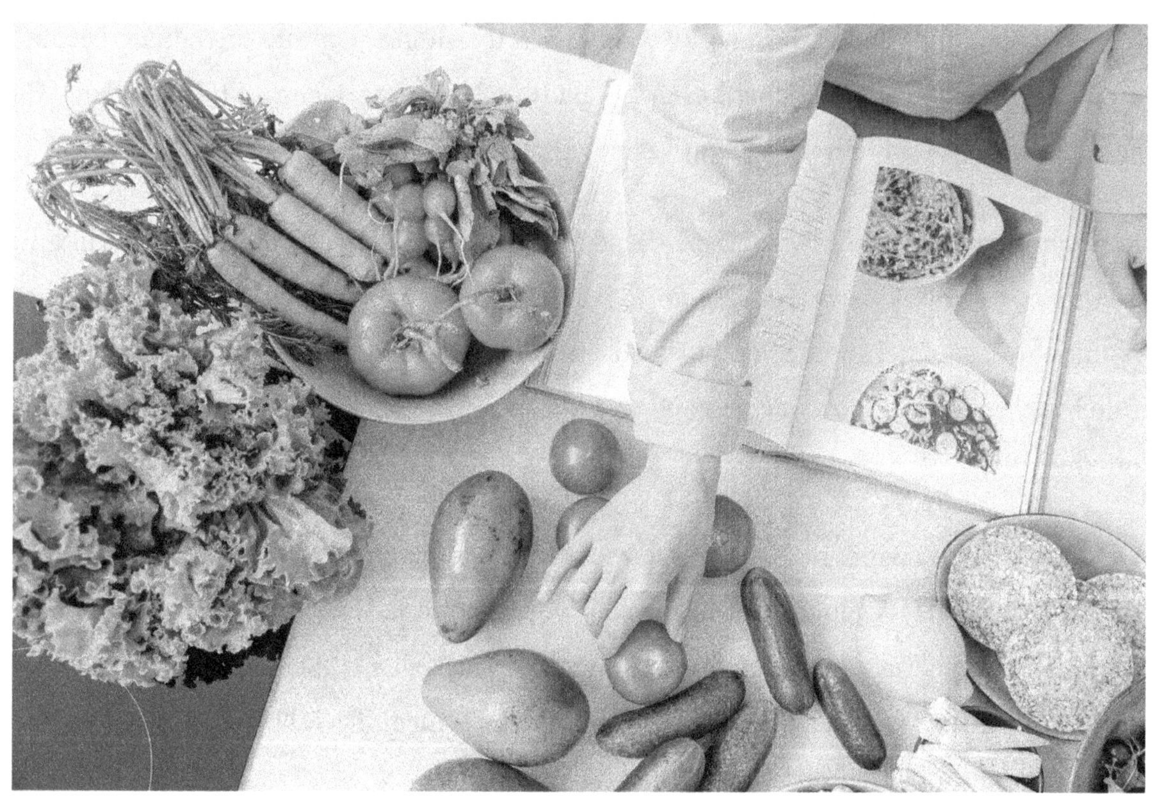

In today's fast-paced world, where stress and unhealthy habits are common, the number of people with chronic diseases, such as inflammatory conditions, has hit scary highs. This detailed guide will go into great detail about inflammatory diseases, including their various types, causes, symptoms, and most importantly, ways to prevent them that can help people live better, more fulfilling lives.

What are Inflammatory Diseases:

Inflammatory diseases are a group of long-term health conditions that cause inflammation to stay in various parts of the body. Chronic inflammation can last for months or even years, damaging tissues and organs. Acute inflammation, on the other hand, is a normal reaction to an injury or infection.

Inflammatory diseases occur when the body's immune system mistakenly attacks its own tissues. This reaction, called inflammation, is normally a defense against infections or injuries. However, in inflammatory diseases, this process happens unnecessarily, leading to pain, redness, swelling, and heat in the affected areas.

One common example is arthritis, where inflammation targets the joints, causing stiffness and pain. Rheumatoid arthritis, a specific type, involves the immune system attacking the lining of the joints. Another example is inflammatory bowel disease (IBD), which includes conditions like Crohn's disease and ulcerative colitis, where inflammation affects the digestive tract, leading to symptoms like abdominal pain, diarrhea, and weight loss.

Inflammation can also affect the skin, as seen in conditions like psoriasis, where skin cells multiply too quickly, causing red, scaly patches. In asthma, inflammation narrows the airways, making it difficult to breathe. Lupus, another inflammatory disease, can impact multiple organs, including the skin, joints, and kidneys, causing a range of symptoms from fatigue to organ damage.

The exact cause of these diseases isn't always clear, but genetics and environmental factors play significant roles. Stress, infections, and certain lifestyle choices, such as smoking or poor diet, can also trigger or worsen inflammation.

Managing inflammatory diseases often involves medications to reduce inflammation and suppress the immune system. Lifestyle changes, like a balanced diet and regular exercise, can help manage symptoms. In some cases, doctors may recommend specific treatments, such as physical therapy for arthritis or dietary adjustments for IBD.
While there is no cure for most inflammatory diseases, understanding their nature helps in managing them effectively, improving the quality of life for those affected.

Various Kinds of Diseases That Increase The Risk of Inflammation:

Several diseases increase the risk of inflammation by causing the immune system to react excessively. These include:

1. Arthritis: There are different types of arthritis, but the most common are osteoarthritis and rheumatoid arthritis. Osteoarthritis occurs when the protective cartilage that cushions the ends of the bones wears down over time, leading to joint inflammation and pain. Rheumatoid arthritis is an autoimmune disease where the immune system attacks the lining of the joints, causing painful swelling and potential joint damage.

*2. **Inflammatory Bowel Disease (IBD):*** This group includes Crohn's disease and ulcerative colitis. Both conditions involve chronic inflammation of the digestive tract. Crohn's disease can affect any part of the gastrointestinal tract, while ulcerative colitis is limited to the colon and rectum. Symptoms include abdominal pain, diarrhea, and weight loss.

*3. **Asthma:*** This chronic disease affects the airways in the lungs. When exposed to triggers like pollen, dust, or smoke, the airways become inflamed and narrow, making it difficult to breathe. Common symptoms include wheezing, shortness of breath, and coughing.

*4. **Psoriasis:*** This skin condition speeds up the life cycle of skin cells, causing cells to build up rapidly on the surface. These extra skin cells form scales and red patches that are often itchy and sometimes painful. Psoriasis is thought to be related to an immune system problem.

*5. **Lupus:*** This autoimmune disease can affect many parts of the body, including the skin, joints, kidneys, and brain. The immune system attacks its own tissues, causing widespread inflammation and damage. Symptoms vary but can include fatigue, joint pain, skin rashes, and fever.

*6. **Multiple Sclerosis (MS):*** In MS, the immune system attacks the protective covering of nerve fibers, causing inflammation and damage to the central nervous system. This disrupts communication between the brain and the rest of the body, leading to symptoms like numbness, weakness, balance issues, and cognitive changes.

*7. **Cardiovascular Diseases:*** Conditions like atherosclerosis, where plaque builds up inside the arteries, can cause inflammation. This buildup can lead to heart attacks and strokes. Chronic inflammation in the arteries plays a significant role in the development and progression of these diseases.

8. *Diabetes:* Particularly type 2 diabetes is linked to chronic inflammation. High blood sugar levels can lead to inflammatory responses in the body, which in turn can cause various complications, including damage to the heart, blood vessels, eyes, kidneys, and nerves.

Understanding these diseases helps in managing inflammation and improving overall health. Treatment often includes medications to control inflammation and lifestyle changes to reduce triggers.

What Causes Inflammatory Diseases?

Inflammatory diseases occur when the body's immune system reacts abnormally, causing inflammation. Here are some common causes:

1. *Autoimmune Reactions:* In some cases, the immune system mistakenly attacks the body's own tissues. This is seen in diseases like rheumatoid arthritis, lupus, and multiple sclerosis. The exact reasons for these reactions are not always clear, but they may involve genetic and environmental factors.

2. *Infections:* Bacteria, viruses, and other pathogens can trigger inflammation as the body tries to fight off these invaders. Sometimes, the immune response continues even after the infection is gone, leading to chronic inflammation. Examples include chronic hepatitis and certain types of arthritis triggered by infections.

3. *Genetics:* Some people are genetically predisposed to inflammatory diseases. If you have a family history of conditions like Crohn's disease, psoriasis, or rheumatoid arthritis, you may be more likely to develop these diseases.

4. *Environmental Factors:* Exposure to certain environmental factors can increase the risk of inflammatory diseases. This includes pollutants, chemicals, and allergens. For instance, smoking and exposure to pollutants can increase the risk of inflammatory lung diseases like asthma.

5. *Diet and Lifestyle:* Poor diet, lack of exercise, and obesity can contribute to inflammation. Diets high in sugar, unhealthy fats, and processed foods can promote inflammatory responses. Excess weight can put extra stress on the body's tissues, leading to conditions like osteoarthritis.

6. *Stress:* Chronic stress can weaken the immune system and lead to inflammation. Stress triggers the release of hormones that can cause the immune system to overreact, leading to or worsening inflammatory diseases.

7. *Injuries:* Physical injuries, such as cuts, sprains, or broken bones, can cause temporary inflammation as the body repairs itself. Sometimes, this inflammation can become chronic if the injury does not heal properly or if there is repeated trauma to the same area.

8. *Age:* As people age, their immune system may become less efficient, leading to increased inflammation. This is why older adults are more prone to inflammatory diseases like arthritis.

9. *Hormonal Changes:* Hormonal imbalances or changes can trigger inflammation. This is often seen in autoimmune diseases which are more common in women, possibly linked to hormonal factors.

10. *Allergies:* Allergic reactions can cause inflammation. When the immune system reacts to harmless substances like pollen, food, or pet dander, it can cause conditions like asthma, eczema, or allergic rhinitis.

Understanding these causes helps in preventing and managing inflammatory diseases. Making healthy lifestyle choices, avoiding known triggers, and seeking medical advice when needed can reduce the risk and impact of these conditions. To

Typical Symptoms of Inflammatory Diseases:

Inflammatory conditions can cause a variety of symptoms, depending on the specific disease and the part of the body affected. Here are some typical symptoms:

1. Pain: This is a common symptom of many inflammatory conditions. It can be sharp or dull and may occur in joints, muscles, or other affected areas. For example, arthritis often causes joint pain.

2. Swelling: Inflammation often leads to swelling in the affected area. This happens because the body's immune response increases blood flow to the area, bringing more white blood cells to fight off potential threats.

3. Redness: The increased blood flow can also cause the skin over the affected area to become red and warm to the touch.

4. Heat: Inflamed areas may feel warm due to increased blood flow. This is another sign that the body is responding to inflammation.

5. Stiffness: Joints or muscles affected by inflammation may feel stiff, making it difficult to move them. This is common in conditions like arthritis.

6. Fatigue: Many inflammatory conditions cause general fatigue or tiredness. The body's effort to fight inflammation can be exhausting, leading to a feeling of constant tiredness.

7. Loss of Function: Inflammation can limit the normal function of the affected area. For instance, inflamed joints may not move as easily, and inflamed muscles might be weaker.

8. Fever: Sometimes, inflammation can cause a fever. This is the body's way of trying to kill off any harmful invaders by creating a less favorable environment for them.

9. General Malaise: This is a feeling of overall discomfort, unease, or illness. It often accompanies chronic inflammatory conditions and can affect daily life.

10. Specific Symptoms Depending on the Condition:

- Asthma: Inflammation of the airways can cause shortness of breath, wheezing, and coughing.

- Psoriasis: Inflammation of the skin leads to red, scaly patches that can be itchy or painful.

- Inflammatory Bowel Disease (IBD): This includes Crohn's disease and ulcerative colitis, which cause symptoms like abdominal pain, diarrhea, weight loss, and sometimes blood in the stool.

- Lupus: This can cause a wide range of symptoms, including joint pain, skin rashes, fatigue, and kidney problems.

11. Loss of Appetite and Weight Loss: Chronic inflammation, especially in diseases like IBD, can reduce appetite and lead to weight loss.

These symptoms can vary widely depending on the specific inflammatory condition and its severity. If you experience persistent or severe symptoms, it's important to seek medical advice for proper diagnosis and treatment.

12. Headaches: Some inflammatory conditions, such as those affecting the sinuses or the brain (like certain types of vasculitis), can result in severe pain, disability, and other complications due to the inflammation and swelling of blood vessels and tissues in affected areas.

Steps to Take to Prevent Inflammatory Diseases:

a) Eating well: Eating a meal that reduces inflammation can greatly lower the chance and severity of these conditions. Fruits, veggies, whole grains, lean meats, and healthy fats are some of the best whole foods to eat. Reduce the amount of processed foods, refined sugars, and whole fats you eat. These foods cause inflammation.

b) Daily Exercise: Being active daily can help lower inflammation, improve the immune system, and keep you healthy in general. You should try to do a mix of cardio, muscle training, and flexibility routines.

c) Effective Stress Management: Long-term stress makes inflammation worse. As a way to relax and improve your general health, try stress-relieving activities like yoga, meditation, deep breathing, or sports.

d) Getting Enough Sleep: Getting enough good sleep is very important for keeping your immune system in check and lowering inflammation. Aim to sleep for 7 to 8 hours straight every night.

e) Avoiding Smoking and Limiting Alcohol Intake: Smoking and drinking too much alcohol make inflammation worse and raise the risk of getting inflammatory diseases. Stop smoking and drink booze in small amounts, if at all.

f) Maintaining Healthy Body Weight: Being overweight makes inflammation worse. A balanced weight can be achieved and maintained by eating well and working out regularly.

Inflammatory diseases are hard to beat, but education and taking steps to prevent them are very helpful. People can take charge of their health and lessen the effects of these long-term conditions by learning about the various types, their causes, and their symptoms, as well as by changing their lifestyles to fight inflammation. Remember that even small changes to your food, exercise, and how you deal with stress can have big effects. Following the recommendations of this guide will help you to lead a life without chronic inflammation, where health and energy thrive.

EAT WELL

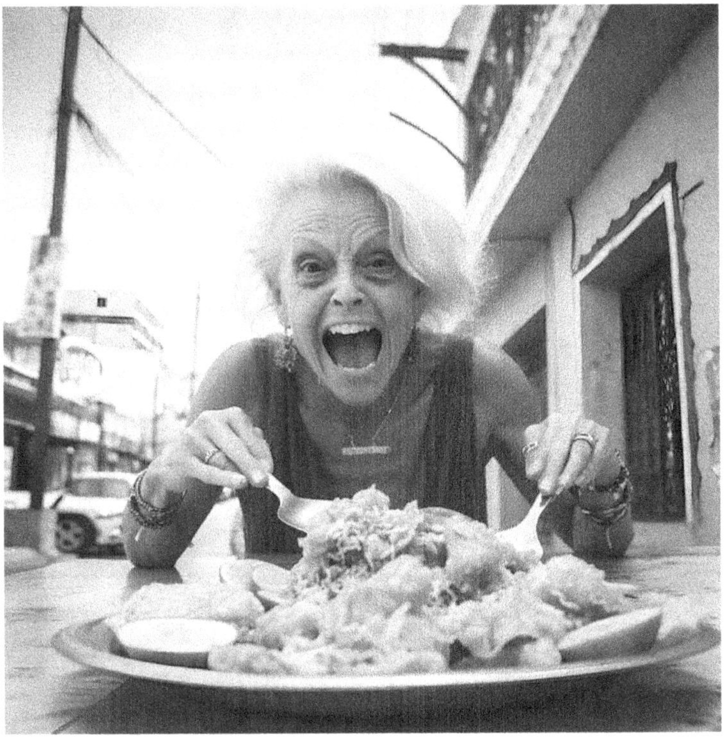

GET ENOUGH SLEEP

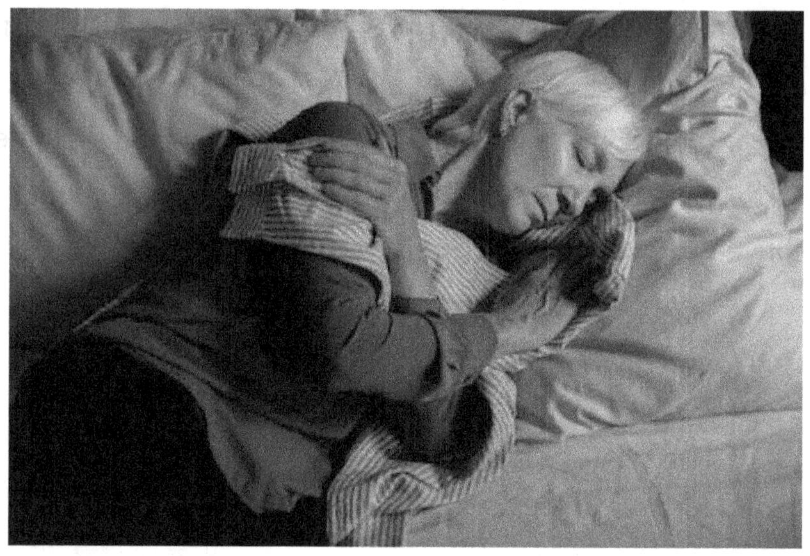

EXERCISE REGULARLY

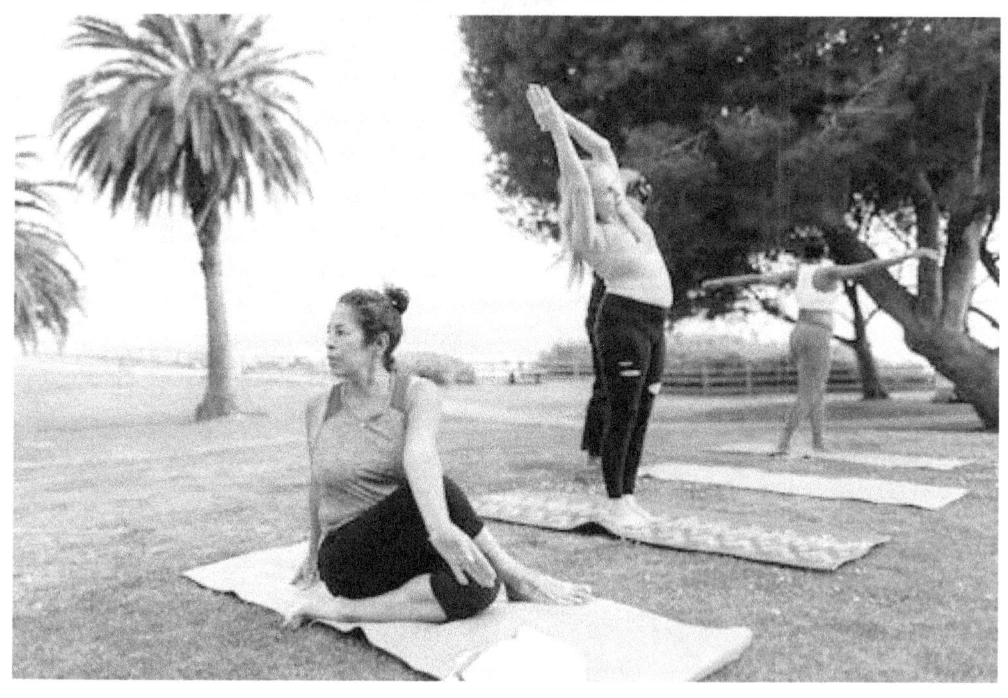

One of the most effective ways to support optimal health and control the symptoms of chronic inflammatory disorders is to adopt an anti-inflammatory diet. You can give your body the nourishment it needs to flourish by including certain meals in your routine and avoiding others that cause inflammation. In this guide, we'll look at what to eat and what not to eat to help you on your path to perfect health.

Foods to Eat:

1. Fruits and Vegetables: Because they are high in phytochemicals and antioxidants that reduce inflammation, pile your plate high with various fruits and vegetables. Cruciferous veggies, colorful peppers, berries, and leafy greens are all great options. To optimize nutrient intake, aim for variety.

2. Healthy Fats:

Include foods like avocados, olive oil, nut, and seeds in your diet as sources of healthy fats. Essential omega-3 fatty acids, which have strong anti-inflammatory effects, are found in these foods. Furthermore, omega-3-rich fatty fish like sardines, mackerel, and salmon have potential health benefits.

3. *Whole Grains:* Refined grains should be avoided for whole grains like quinoa, brown rice, and whole wheat bread. In addition to other nutrients, fiber present in whole grains helps control blood sugar levels and minimize inflammation.

4. *Lean Proteins:* Choose tofu, skinless chicken, fish, and lentils as your lean protein sources. These meals supply the necessary amino acids without the extra saturated fats that cause inflammation, which are present in red meat.

5. *Herbs and Spices:* Use anti-inflammatory herbs and spices like turmeric, ginger, garlic, cinnamon, and rosemary to enhance the flavor of your food. These ingredients have potent anti-inflammatory properties in addition to giving your food depth.

Foods to Avoid:

1. *Processed and Refined Foods:* Cut back on, or completely cut out, these items from your diet. These include pastries, white bread, quick meals, and sweet snacks. These meals frequently have high concentrations of added sugars, unhealthy fats, and preservatives, all of which worsen inflammation.

2. *Trans Fats:* Steer clear of meals high in trans fats, like margarine, packaged snacks, and fried foods. Trans fats raise the risk of heart disease in addition to inflaming the body.

3. *Sugary Drinks:* Limit your intake of fruit juices, energy drinks, and sugar-filled sodas. These drinks have a lot of added sugar, which may trigger inflammation and other health problems.

4. *Excessive Alcohol:* Although moderate alcohol use may offer certain health benefits, consuming too much alcohol can cause inflammation and harm various organs. Either cut back on your alcohol intake or stay away from it completely.

5. *High-salt Foods:* Cut back on your intake of foods high in salt, such as canned soups, processed meats, and fast food. High sodium levels have been linked to inflammation and increased blood pressure risk.

In summary, you may make a big difference in your health and well-being by eating an anti-inflammatory diet and paying attention to what you put in your mouth. Lean proteins, whole grains, healthy fats, and a rainbow of fruits and vegetables can help you provide your body with the nutrition it needs to function while lowering inflammation. Avoid or limit trans fats, sugary drinks, processed and refined foods, high-sodium foods, and excessive alcohol consumption at the same time. Recall that even minor dietary adjustments can have a big impact on your general health. On your path to optimal health, nourish your body with the proper foods and embrace the transformative potential of an anti-inflammatory diet.

Benefits of Following an Anti-Inflammatory Diet Regimen

Seniors who follow an anti-inflammatory diet can reap the following main benefits:

1. *Lower Inflammation:* Alzheimer's, heart disease, arthritis, and other diseases associated with aging are all linked to chronic inflammation. Inflammation in the body can be reduced by eating a diet high in fruits, vegetables, whole grains, lean meats, and healthy fats like omega-3 fatty acids. This may help lessen the symptoms associated with various inflammatory diseases.

*2. **Better Joint Health:*** Due to diseases like arthritis, seniors frequently experience joint stiffness and pain. Antioxidant-rich foods, such as berries and leafy greens, can provide relief from joint inflammation and possibly even slow down the advancement of joint-related conditions.

*3. **Heart Health:*** Foods that can promote heart health, such as nuts, seeds, olive oil, and oily fish high in omega-3 fatty acids, are often included in an anti-inflammatory diet. For seniors who are more vulnerable to heart-related conditions, these meals can help lower cholesterol, lessen the risk of blood clots, and enhance overall cardiovascular function.

*4. **Cognitive Function:*** Research has connected deterioration in cognitive function to long-term inflammation in the body. Seniors can enhance cognitive performance and lower their risk of dementia and Alzheimer's disease by eating anti-inflammatory diseases foods such as fatty fish, berries, and leafy greens high in antioxidants and omega-3 fatty acids.

*5. **Digestive Health:*** A diet high in whole foods and fiber-rich fruits and vegetables can help maintain a healthy gut microbiota by reducing inflammation. This may improve digestion, increase the absorption of nutrients, and lower the risk of digestive problems that seniors frequently experience, like bloating and constipation.

*6. **Weight Management:*** Because of their slowed metabolisms and decreased levels of physical activity, seniors may find it more difficult to maintain a healthy weight. An anti-inflammatory diet rich in whole, nutrient-dense foods can lessen cravings for unhealthy processed foods, assist control of appetite, and promote weight management—all of which are crucial to older persons' general health and well-being.

Seniors may experience these benefits, which can enhance general health, vitality, and quality of life as they age, by adopting an anti-inflammatory diet into their lifestyle. Before making major dietary changes, seniors should speak with a doctor or a qualified dietitian to make sure their unique nutritional requirements and medical problems are taken into consideration.

FOODDS THAT REDUCE OR COMBAT INFLAMMATION

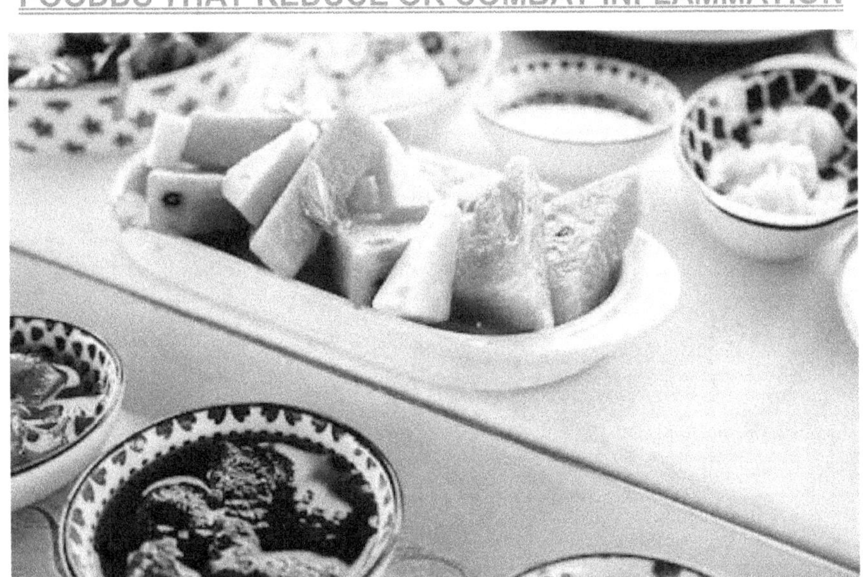

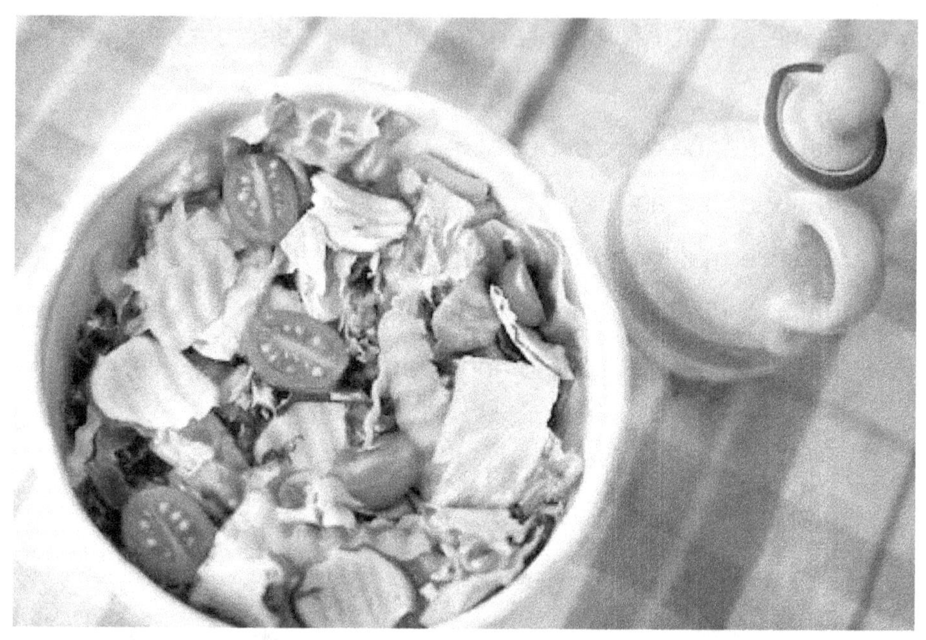

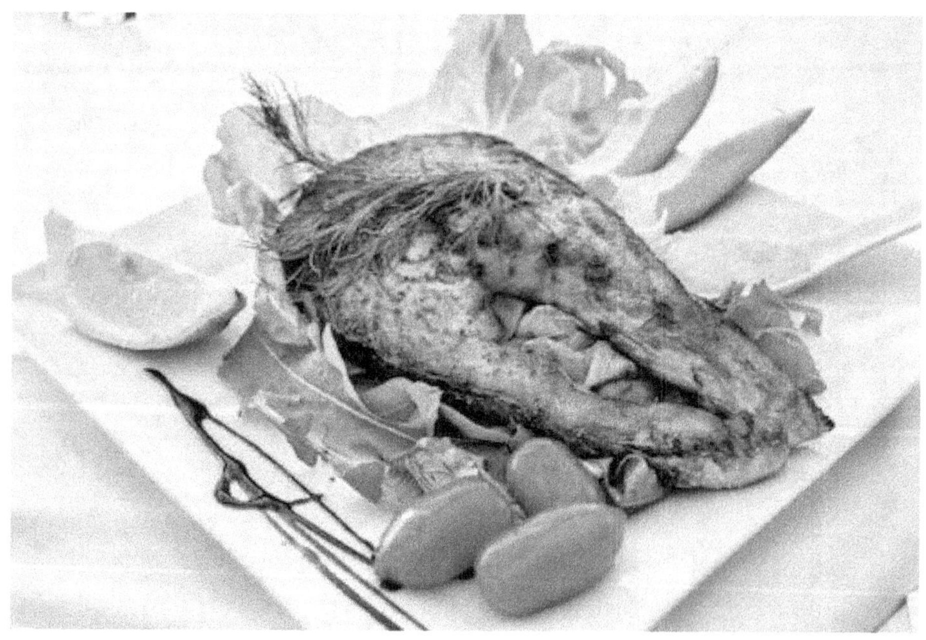

Following an anti-inflammatory diet regimen involves making specific dietary choices to reduce inflammation in the body. Here are the key steps to following an anti-inflammatory diet:

1. Focus on Whole Foods: Base your diet on whole, unprocessed foods such as fruits, vegetables, whole grains, nuts, seeds, and legumes. These foods are rich in antioxidants, vitamins, minerals, and fiber that can help combat inflammation.

2. Eat Omega-3 Fatty Acids: Incorporate foods rich in omega-3 fatty acids, such as fatty fish (salmon, mackerel, and sardines), flaxseeds, chia seeds, and walnuts. Omega-3 fatty acids have anti-inflammatory properties and are beneficial for heart and brain health.

3. Include Healthy Fats: Opt for healthy fats like olive oil, avocado, and nuts instead of saturated and trans fats found in processed foods. These fats can help reduce inflammation in the body and support overall health.

4. Limit Sugar and Refined Carbohydrates: Reduce your intake of added sugars, sugary beverages, processed snacks, and refined carbohydrates like white bread and pastries. These foods can trigger inflammation and spike blood sugar levels.

5. Avoid Processed Foods: Minimize your consumption of processed and packaged foods that are high in unhealthy fats, sugar, and additives. These foods can promote inflammation in the body and contribute to various health issues.

6. *Spices and Herbs:* Incorporate anti-inflammatory spices and herbs like turmeric, ginger, garlic, cinnamon, and rosemary into your meals. These ingredients have potent anti-inflammatory properties and can add flavor to your dishes.

7. *Stay Hydrated:* Drink an adequate amount of water throughout the day to stay hydrated and support overall bodily functions. Herbal teas and water with lemon can also be beneficial.

8. *Maintain a Balanced Diet:* Ensure that your meals are well-balanced and include a variety of foods from various food groups to meet your nutritional needs. Include a variety of colorful fruits and vegetables to benefit from a range of antioxidants.

9. *Listen to Your Body:* Pay attention to how your body responds to certain foods. If you notice any adverse reactions or sensitivities, consider eliminating those foods from your diet to reduce inflammation and improve overall health.

10. *Consult a Professional:* If you have specific health conditions or dietary concerns, consider consulting a healthcare provider or a registered dietitian who can provide personalized guidance tailored to your individual needs and health goals when following an anti-inflammatory diet regimen.

By following these guidelines and making mindful food choices, you can adopt an anti-inflammatory diet regimen that supports overall health, reduces inflammation, and promotes well-being.

When shopping for an anti-inflammatory diet to help combat diseases and promote overall health, here are 20 healthy ingredients and foods to include on your shopping list:

1. Fatty Fish: Salmon, mackerel, sardines, and trout are rich in omega-3 fatty acids, which have anti-inflammatory properties.

2. Berries: Blueberries, strawberries, raspberries, and blackberries are packed with antioxidants that help fight inflammation.

3. Leafy Greens: Spinach, kale, Swiss chard, and collard greens contain vitamins, minerals, and antioxidants that combat inflammation.

4. Turmeric: A spice with potent anti-inflammatory effects due to its active compound curcumin.

5. Ginger: Contains gingerol, which has anti-inflammatory and antioxidant properties.

6. Nuts and Seeds: Almonds, walnuts, flaxseeds, chia seeds, and hemp seeds are rich in healthy fats and antioxidants.

7. Olive Oil: Extra virgin olive oil is a source of monounsaturated fats and antioxidants that combat inflammation.

8. Avocado: Rich in monounsaturated fats and fiber, avocados help reduce inflammation.

9. Broccoli: Packed with sulforaphane, a compound that has anti-inflammatory effects.

10. Tomatoes: High in lycopene, an antioxidant that reduces inflammation and can help protect against certain diseases.

11. Green Tea: Contains polyphenols that have anti-inflammatory and antioxidant effects.

12. Whole Grains: Choose whole grains like quinoa, brown rice, oats, and barley for fiber and nutrients that fight inflammation.

13. Legumes: Beans, lentils, and chickpeas are rich in fiber and plant-based protein, which can help reduce inflammation.

14. Garlic: Contains sulfur compounds with potent anti-inflammatory properties.

15. **Yogurt:** Opt for low-fat or Greek yogurt with probiotics that support gut health and reduce inflammation.

16. Tart Cherries: Known for their anti-inflammatory properties and potential benefits for reducing muscle soreness.

17. Bell Peppers: High in vitamin C and antioxidants that combat inflammation.

18. Cinnamon: Contains antioxidants and has anti-inflammatory effects

19. Carrots: Rich in beta-carotene, which converts to vitamin A in the body and has anti-inflammatory properties.

20. Dark Chocolate (70% cocoa or higher): Contains antioxidants such as flavonoids that help fight inflammation and improve heart health.

By including these healthy ingredients in your shopping list and incorporating them into your meals regularly, you can create a well-rounded anti-inflammatory diet to support your health and well-being. Remember to vary your choices and opt for whole, minimally processed foods to maximize the benefits of an anti-inflammatory diet.

When the proper anti-inflammatory diet regimen is not adopted, individuals may experience various complications related to inflammatory diseases. Chronic inflammation is associated with numerous health issues, and neglecting dietary guidelines aimed at reducing inflammation can exacerbate these conditions and lead to further complications. One of the significant complications of not following an anti-inflammatory diet is the perpetuation of inflammatory responses in the body. Inflammation is a natural and necessary process in response to injury or infection.

However, chronic inflammation, engendered by poor dietary choices, can lead to a range of health problems. Without the right nutrients to support an anti-inflammatory response, the body's immune system may become overactive, triggering a chain of inflammatory reactions that can damage healthy cells and tissues. This can worsen the symptoms of inflammatory diseases such as rheumatoid arthritis, inflammatory bowel disease, or even cardiovascular condition

Moreover, a diet lacking in anti-inflammatory foods can contribute to the worsening of age-related diseases. Conditions like Alzheimer's, cardiovascular disease, and diabetes have links to chronic inflammation. By not consuming foods rich in antioxidants, omega-3 fatty acids, and other anti-inflammatory compounds, individuals may be at a higher risk of developing these diseases or experiencing more severe symptoms if they already have them.

Another complication of ignoring an anti-inflammatory diet is the potential impact on joint health. Arthritis, both osteoarthritis and rheumatoid arthritis, can be aggravated by inflammation. Without the anti-inflammatory properties of certain foods, joint pain, stiffness, and swelling can worsen. This may limit mobility and decrease the quality of life for individuals living with these conditions.

Furthermore, the absence of an anti-inflammatory diet can negatively affect cardiovascular health. Chronic inflammation is a significant risk factor for heart disease. Without the protective effects of foods like fatty fish, nuts, olive oil, and fruits and vegetables rich in antioxidants, individuals may experience heightened levels of inflammation in the arteries, leading to atherosclerosis, blood clots, or other cardiovascular complications.

Additionally, cognitive function may be compromised if an anti-inflammatory diet regimen is not adopted. Studies have shown that chronic inflammation is associated with cognitive decline and neurodegenerative diseases like Alzheimer's. Without the brain-boosting nutrients found in foods like berries, leafy greens, and fatty fish, individuals may be more susceptible to memory problems, decreased cognitive abilities, and a higher risk of developing dementia.

In summary, the complications of not following an anti-inflammatory diet can be far-reaching and detrimental to one's overall health and well-being. By neglecting to incorporate anti-inflammatory foods into their diet, individuals may worsen the symptoms of inflammatory diseases, increase the risk of age-related conditions, compromise joint and cardiovascular health, and impair cognitive function. Adopting an anti-inflammatory diet is crucial for managing inflammation, preventing disease, and promoting longevity and vitality.

For an anti-inflammatory disease diet, meal planning means choosing and making foods that are specifically designed to lower inflammation in the body. This method not only helps control the symptoms of inflammatory conditions, but it also has many other health and wellness benefits.

Benefits of Meal Planning for an Anti-Inflammatory Disease Diet:

1. *Consistency:* Planning meals helps people stick to a controlled and regular eating schedule. It's easier to stick to an anti-inflammatory diet plan when you plan your meals ahead of time and prepare your meals ahead of time.

2. *Balanced Nutrition:* People can make sure they are getting a well-rounded and balanced diet by planning their meals ahead of time. They can meet their nutritional needs and improve their health by eating a range of nutrient-dense foods, like fruits, vegetables, whole grains, lean proteins, and healthy fats.

3. *Portion Control:* Planning meals helps you keep track of how much you eat, which is important for keeping your weight in check and not eating too much. By planning their meals ahead of time, people can avoid eating too many calories, which can lead to inflammation and other health problems.

4. *Time-Saving:* Making plans for meals ahead of time can help you find time during the busy weekdays. People can spend less time making meals every day by preparing items ahead of time, cooking in bulk, or having meals ready to go. This makes it easier to stick to a healthy eating plan.

5. *Saves money:* Planning meals can also save you money. People can save money by buying items in bulk or when they are on sale and reducing food waste by making a shopping list based on the meals they plan to eat.

6. *Diverse and Varied Diet:* Planning meals helps you eat a wide variety of foods, which is important for getting all the nutrients and antioxidants that fight inflammation. Eating healthy can be more fun and sustainable if you try new recipes and eat foods from different food groups.

7. *Improved Digestion:* An anti-inflammatory diet can help gut health and improve digestion by choosing foods that are easy on the digestive system and high in fiber. This may be good for your general health and may help people with digestive problems that are caused by inflammation.

8. *Long-Term Health Benefits:* Planning your meals can help your health in the long run by helping you eat a diet that lowers inflammation. By mitigating chronic inflammation, people may lower their risk of developing inflammatory diseases like gout, heart disease, and other health issues that come with getting older.

7-Day Meal Plan for Anti-Inflammatory Diseases Diet

Here is a sample 7-day anti-inflammatory diseases meal plan to help you get started on incorporating anti-inflammatory foods into your diet:

Day 1:

- ***Breakfast:*** Greek yogurt topped with berries and a sprinkle of chia seeds.

- ***Lunch:*** Quinoa salad with mixed greens, cherry tomatoes, cucumbers, and grilled chicken.

- ***Dinner:*** Baked salmon with a side of steamed broccoli and quinoa.

Day 2:

- *Breakfast:* Oatmeal with walnuts, cinnamon, and sliced strawberries.

- *Lunch:* Lentil soup with a side of mixed green salad.

- *Dinner:* Stir-fried tofu with mixed vegetables and brown rice.

Day 3:

- *Breakfast:* Whole grain toast with avocado mash and a poached egg.

- *Lunch:* Chickpea salad with diced bell peppers, red onion, parsley, and a lemon vinaigrette.

- *Dinner:* Turkey chili with black beans, tomatoes, and bell peppers.

Day 4:

- *Breakfast:* Smoothie with spinach, banana, almond milk, and a spoon of almond butter.

- *Lunch:* Grilled vegetable and hummus wrap with a side of baby carrots.

- *Dinner:* Baked chicken breast with roasted sweet potatoes and asparagus.

Day 5:

- *Breakfast:* Buckwheat pancakes topped with Greek yogurt and sliced peaches.

- *Lunch:* Quinoa-stuffed bell peppers with a side of mixed green salad.

- *Dinner:* Zucchini noodles with homemade tomato sauce and lean ground turkey.

Day 6:

- *Breakfast:* Chia seed pudding with fresh fruit and a drizzle of honey.

- *Lunch:* Lentil and kale salad with cherry tomatoes and a balsamic vinaigrette.

- *Dinner:* Grilled shrimp skewers with roasted Brussels sprouts and wild rice.

Day 7:

- *Breakfast:* An acai bowl topped with granola, coconut flakes, and mixed berries.

- *Lunch:* Tuna salad with mixed greens, cucumber, and avocado.

- *Dinner:* Baked cod with a side of quinoa and sautéed spinach.

These meals can be repeated or adapted week after week and incorporate your favorite anti-inflammatory foods, trying new recipes, and ensuring you have a variety of fruits, vegetables, whole grains, lean proteins, and healthy fats.

Remember to stay hydrated throughout the day, snack on nuts, seeds, and fruits if needed, and consult with a healthcare provider or a nutritionist to personalize this meal plan to suit your individual dietary needs and preferences. Following an anti-inflammatory diet consistently can help in managing inflammatory diseases and promoting overall health and well-being. Enjoy your meals!

10 Delicious Breakfast Recipes

Here are 10 anti-inflammatory breakfast recipes with ingredients, preparation methods, quantities, nutritional value, and estimated cooking times:

1. Berry Chia Seed Pudding:

Ingredients:

- 1/4 cup chia seeds

- 1 cup almond milk

- 1/2 teaspoon vanilla extract

- Mixed berries (blueberries, strawberries, raspberries)

Preparation: Mix chia seeds, almond milk, and vanilla extract in a jar. Let it sit in the fridge overnight. In the morning, top with mixed berries.

Nutritional Value: Rich in omega-3 fatty acids, fiber, antioxidants, and vitamins.

Cooking Time: 5 minutes of prep time; overnight to set.

2. Turmeric Quinoa Breakfast Bowl:

Ingredients:

- 1/2 cup cooked quinoa

- 1/4 teaspoon turmeric

- 1 tablespoon honey

- Sliced almonds and dried apricots

Preparation: Mix cooked quinoa with turmeric and honey. Top with sliced almonds and dried apricots.

Nutritional Value: High in protein, fiber, anti-inflammatory properties from turmeric, and essential minerals.

Cooking Time: 15 minutes to cook quinoa; 5 minutes prep time.

3. Avocado and Egg Toast:

Ingredients:

- 1 slice whole grain bread

- 1/2 ripe avocado

- 1 poached egg

- Chili flakes and sea salt

Preparation: Toast bread, mash avocado on top, place poached egg, sprinkle with chili flakes and sea salt.

Nutritional Value: Good source of healthy fats, protein, fiber, and vitamins.

Cooking Time: 10 minutes to poach egg; 5 minutes prep time.

4. Spinach and Feta Omelete:

Ingredients:

- 3 eggs

- Handful of fresh spinach

- 1/4 cup crumbled feta cheese

- Salt and pepper to taste

Preparation: Whisk eggs, add spinach and feta, season with salt and pepper, and cook like an omelet.

Nutritional Value: High in protein, iron, calcium, vitamins, and antioxidants from spinach.

Cooking Time: 10 minutes.

5. Coconut Mango Smoothie Bowl:

Ingredients:

- 1/2 cup coconut milk
- 1/2 cup frozen mango chunks
- 1 banana
- Toppings: shredded coconut, chia seeds, sliced almonds

Preparation: Blend coconut milk, mango, and banana until smooth. Top with coconut, chia seeds, and almonds.

Nutritional Value: Provides fiber, healthy fats, vitamins, and minerals.

Cooking Time: 5 minutes.

6. Greek Yogurt Parfait:

Ingredients:

- 1 cup Greek yogurt
- 1/4 cup granola
- Mixed berries
- Honey

Preparation: Layer Greek yogurt, granola, and berries in a glass. Drizzle honey on top.

Nutritional Value: High in protein, probiotics, fiber, and antioxidants.

Cooking Time: 5 minutes.

7. Almond Butter Banana Smoothie:

Ingredients:

- 1 ripe banana
- 1 tablespoon almond butter
- 1 cup almond milk
- Handful of spinach

Preparation: Blend banana, almond butter, almond milk, and spinach until smooth.

Nutritional Value: Rich in potassium, healthy fats, vitamins, and antioxidants.

Cooking Time: 5 minutes.

8. Matcha Green Tea Overnight Oats:

Ingredients:

- 1/2 cup rolled oats
- 1 teaspoon matcha powder
- 1 tablespoon honey
- Almond milk

Preparation: Mix oats, matcha, honey, and almond milk in a jar. Keep in the fridge overnight.

Nutritional Value: Provides fiber, antioxidants, energy, and vitamins.

Cooking Time: Overnight to set.

9. Sweet Potato and Kale Breakfast Hash:

Ingredients:

- 1 sweet potato, diced
- Handful of kale, chopped
- 1/2 red onion, diced
- Olive oil

Preparation: Sauté sweet potato, kale, and onion in olive oil until cooked through.

Nutritional Value: High in vitamins, fiber, antioxidants, and anti-inflammatory properties.

Cooking Time: 15 minutes.

10. Blueberry Almond Butter Toast:

Ingredients:

- 2 slices whole grain bread
- Almond butter
- Fresh blueberries
- Drizzle of honey

Preparation: Toast bread, spread almond butter, top with blueberries, and drizzle honey.

Nutritional Value: Provides protein, healthy fats, antioxidants, and fiber.

Cooking Time: 5 minutes.

These breakfast recipes are not only delicious but also packed with nutrients that can help combat inflammation and promote overall health. Enjoy trying out these flavorful and nourishing meal ideas!

10 Mouthwatering Anti-inflammatory Lunch Recipes

1: Lentil and Vegetable Soup

Ingredients:
- 1 cup dried lentils

- 4 cups vegetable broth

- 1 onion, diced

- 2 carrots, sliced

- 2 celery stalks, diced

- 2 cloves garlic, minced

- 1 tsp turmeric

- Salt and pepper to taste

Preparation:
1. Rinse lentils and place them in a pot with vegetable broth. Bring to a boil.

2. Add onion, carrots, celery, garlic, turmeric, salt, and pepper.

3. Simmer for 25-30 minutes until lentils are tender.

4. Adjust seasoning if needed. Serve hot.

Nutritional Value: High in fiber, plant-based protein, and anti-inflammatory properties.

Cooking Time: Approximately 30 minutes.

2: Salmon and Quinoa Salad

Ingredients:
  - 1 cup cooked quinoa

  - 6 oz grilled salmon, flaked

  - 1 cup cherry tomatoes, halved

  - 1 cucumber, diced

  - 2 tablespoons olive oil

  - 1 tablespoons lemon juice

  - Fresh dill, chopped

Preparation:
  1. In a bowl, combine quinoa, salmon, cherry tomatoes, cucumber, and dill.

  2. In a separate bowl, whisk olive oil and lemon juice. Pour over the salad.

  3. Toss gently to combine. Serve chilled.

Nutritional Value: Rich in omega-3 fatty acids, protein, antioxidants, and essential nutrients.

Cooking Time: 20 minutes for salmon, quinoa prep time excluded.

3: Chickpea and Avocado Wrap

Ingredients:
  - 1 can chickpeas, drained
  - 1 ripe avocado, mashed

  - 1/4 cup diced red onion

  - 1/4 cup chopped cilantro

  - Juice of 1 lime

  - Salt and pepper to taste

  - Whole grain wraps

Preparation:

1. In a bowl, mash chickpeas with avocado, red onion, cilantro, lime juice, salt, and pepper.

2. Spread the mixture on a whole-grain wrap, roll it up, and cut it in half.

3. Serve with a side salad or veggie sticks.

Nutritional Value: High in fiber, healthy fats, plant-based protein, and vitamins.

Cooking Time: Prep time is about 10-15 minutes.

Feel free to try these recipes in your quest for anti-inflammatory lunch options that are both delicious and beneficial for your health.

4: Quinoa-Stuffed Bell Peppers

Ingredients:
- 4 bell peppers, halved and seeds removed
- 1 cup cooked quinoa
- 1 can black beans, rinsed
- 1 cup corn kernels
- 1/2 cup diced tomatoes
- 1/2 teaspoons cumin
- 1/2 teaspoons paprika
- Salt and pepper to taste

Preparation:
1. Preheat oven to 375°F (190°C).

2. In a bowl, mix quinoa, black beans, corn, tomatoes, cumin, paprika, salt, and pepper.

3. Stuff the bell pepper halves with the quinoa mixture.

4. Place peppers in a baking dish, cover with foil and bake for 25-30 minutes.

5. Remove foil and bake for an additional 10 minutes. Serve hot

Nutritional Value: Packed with fiber, protein, antioxidants, and essential nutrients.

Cooking Time: Approximately 40 minutes.

5: Grilled Vegetable Salad with Lemon Tahini Dressing

Ingredients:
- Assorted vegetables (bell peppers, zucchini, eggplant)
- 2 tablespoons olive oil
- Salt and pepper to taste
- 1/4 cup of tahini
- Juice of 1 lemon
- 1 garlic clove, minced
- Water (for thinning dressing)

Preparation:
1. Toss vegetables with olive oil, salt, and pepper.
2. Grill vegetables until tender and slightly charred.
3. In a bowl, whisk tahini, lemon juice, garlic, and water to desired consistency.
4. Arrange grilled vegetables on a plate, drizzle with dressing, and serve.

Nutritional Value: Rich in vitamins, minerals, antioxidants, and healthy fats.

Cooking Time: Grill time varies based on vegetable selection

6: Tofu and Vegetable Stir-Fry

Ingredients:

- 1 block of firm tofu, cubed
- 2 cups mixed vegetables (bell peppers, broccoli, snap peas)
- 2 tablespoons soy sauce

- 1 tablespoons sesame oil

- 1 teaspoon grated ginger

- 2 garlic cloves, minced

- Cooked brown rice

Preparation:

1. Heat sesame oil in a pan, add tofu cubes and cook until golden brown.

2. Add mixed vegetables, ginger, garlic, and soy sauce. Stir-fry until vegetables are tender.

3. Serve over brown rice.

Nutritional Value: High in plant-based protein, fiber, vitamins, and antioxidants.

Cooking Time: About 20 minutes.

These additional lunch recipes offer a variety of flavors and nutrients to support an anti-inflammatory diet and promote overall health and well-being. Enjoy these wholesome meals as part of your daily menu

7: Turmeric Chicken Skewers

Ingredients:

- 2 chicken breasts, cut into chunks

- 1 tablespoons olive oil

- 1 teaspoon turmeric

- 1/2 teaspoon cumin

- 1/2 teaspoon paprika

- Salt and pepper to taste

Preparation:

1. In a bowl, mix olive oil, turmeric, cumin, paprika, salt, and pepper.

2. Add chicken chunks and coat well. Marinate for 30 minutes.

3. Thread chicken onto skewers and grill or bake until cooked through.

4. Serve with a side salad or quinoa.

Nutritional Value: Protein-rich, anti-inflammatory spices, and low in saturated fats.

Cooking Time: Grilling time is approximately 15-20 minutes.

8: Sweet Potato and Lentil Shepherd's Pie

Ingredients:

- 2 large sweet potatoes, peeled and cubed

- 1 cup cooked green lentils

- 1 onion, diced

- 2 carrots, diced

- 1 cup peas

- 1 teaspoon thyme

- Salt and pepper to taste

Preparation:

1. Boil sweet potatoes until tender, then mash them.

2. In a skillet, sauté onion and carrots until soft.

3. Add lentils, peas, thyme, salt, and pepper. Cook for 5 minutes.

4. Transfer the lentil mixture to a baking dish, and top with mashed sweet potatoes.

5. Bake at 375°F (190°C) for 20-25 minutes until golden.

Nutritional Value: High in fiber, plant-based protein, vitamins, and minerals.

Cooking Time: Approximately 45 minutes.

9: Mediterranean Quinoa Salad

Ingredients:
- 1 cup cooked quinoa

- 1 can chickpeas, rinsed

- 1 cucumber, diced

- 1 cup cherry tomatoes, halved

- 1/4 cup Kalamata olives, sliced

- Feta cheese, crumbled (optional)

- Fresh parsley, chopped

Preparation:

1. Combine quinoa, chickpeas, cucumber, tomatoes, olives, and parsley in a bowl.

2. Add feta cheese if desired and toss gently.

3. Drizzle with olive oil and lemon juice before serving.

Nutritional Value: Rich in protein, antioxidants, healthy fats, and Mediterranean flavors.

Cooking Time: Approximately 20 minutes for quinoa prep.

10: Spinach and Mushroom Stuffed Chicken Breast

Ingredients:

- 2 chicken breasts
- 1 cup baby spinach
- 1 cup mushrooms, diced
- 2 garlic cloves, minced
- 1/4 cup grated Parmesan cheese
- Salt and pepper to taste

Preparation:

1. Preheat the oven to 375°F (190°C).
2. Pound chicken breasts to flatten. Season with salt and pepper.
3. Sauté spinach, mushrooms, and garlic until wilted. Stir in Parmesan cheese.
4. Spoon the spinach mixture onto the chicken breasts, roll them up, and secure them with toothpicks.
5. Bake for 25-30 minutes until the chicken is cooked through.

Nutritional Value: Protein-packed, low-carb, and loaded with vitamins and minerals.

Cooking Time: Approximately 30 minutes.

These nutritious and flavorful lunch recipes cater to an anti-inflammatory diet, providing a range of options to keep your meals exciting, delicious, and beneficial for your health. Enjoy these wholesome dishes as part of your balanced eating plan!

10 Tantalizing Dinner Recipes for Anti-Inflammatory Diet

1: Baked Salmon with Quinoa and Roasted Vegetables

Ingredients:

- 2 salmon fillets

- 1 cup quinoa

- 1 zucchini, sliced

- 1 red bell pepper, sliced

- 1 tablespoon olive oil

- 1 lemon, sliced

- Salt and pepper to taste

Preparation:

1. Preheat the oven to 400°F (200°C).

2. Season salmon fillets with salt, pepper, and a squeeze of lemon. Place lemon slices on top.

3. Cook quinoa according to package instructions.

4. Toss zucchini and bell pepper with olive oil, salt, and pepper. Roast in the oven for 20-25 minutes.

5. Bake salmon for 15-20 minutes until cooked through.

6. Serve the salmon on a bed of quinoa with roasted vegetables on the side.

Nutritional Value: High in Omega-3 fatty acids, protein, fiber, vitamins, and antioxidants.

Cooking Time: Approximately 30-35 minutes.

2: Lentil and Sweet Potato Curry

Ingredients:

- 1 cup dried lentils
- 2 sweet potatoes, peeled and cubed
- 1 onion, chopped
- 3 garlic cloves, minced
- 1 can of coconut milk
- 2tablespoons of curry powder
- Salt and pepper to taste

Preparation:

1. Cook lentils according to package instructions.
2. In a separate pot, sauté onion and garlic until soft.
3. Add sweet potatoes, curry powder, salt, and pepper. Cook for 5 minutes.
4. Pour in coconut milk and simmer until sweet potatoes are tender.
5. Stir in cooked lentils and adjust seasoning if needed.
6. Serve the curry hot with brown rice or quinoa.

Nutritional Value: Rich in plant-based protein, fiber, complex carbohydrates, and anti-inflammatory spices.

Cooking Time: Approximately 45-50 minutes.

3: Turkey Meatballs with Zucchini Noodles

Ingredients:

- 1 lb of ground turkey

- 2 zucchinis, spiralized

- 1 can diced tomatoes

- 1/4 cup almond flour

- 1 egg

- 2 garlic cloves, minced

- 1 tsp. dried oregano

Preparation:

1. Preheat the oven to 375°F (190°C).

2. In a bowl, mix ground turkey, almond flour, egg, garlic, oregano, salt, and pepper. Form into meatballs.

3. Place the meatballs on a baking sheet and bake for 20-25 minutes.

4. Heat diced tomatoes with garlic, oregano, salt, and pepper in a skillet.

5. Add zucchini noodles and cook for 3-4 minutes until tender.

6. Serve the turkey meatballs on top of the zucchini noodles and tomato sauce.

Nutritional Value: Low-fat protein source, low-carb, high in fiber, vitamins, and minerals.

Cooking Time: Approximately 30-35 minutes.

These dinner recipes provide a nutritious and flavorful way to include anti-inflammatory ingredients in your meals, supporting your health and well-being. Enjoy these wholesome dishes as part of your evening routine!

4. Turmeric Chicken with Quinoa and Roasted Vegetables

Ingredients:

- 2 chicken breasts
- 1 tablespoon turmeric powder
- 1 cup quinoa
- 2 cups mixed vegetables (bell peppers, zucchini, carrots)
- Olive oil
- Salt and pepper to taste

Preparation:

- Marinate chicken breasts with turmeric, salt, and pepper.
- Cook quinoa according to package instructions.
- Toss mixed vegetables with olive oil, salt, and pepper. Roast in the oven at 400°F (200°C) for 20-25 minutes.
- Grill or pan-sear chicken breasts until fully cooked, about 6-8 minutes per side.
- Serve grilled chicken with quinoa and roasted vegetables.

Nutritional Info:

- Calories: 400 per serving
- Protein: 30g
- Carbohydrates: 40g
- Fat: 12g
- Fiber: 8g

5.   Salmon with Garlic Kale and Sweet Potato Mash

Ingredients:

- 2 salmon fillets
- 2 cups kale, chopped
- 2 cloves garlic, minced
- 2 medium sweet potatoes, peeled and diced
- Olive oil
- Salt and pepper to taste

Preparation:

- Season salmon fillets with salt and pepper. Grill or bake until cooked through about 10-12 minutes.
- In a pan, sauté minced garlic in olive oil until fragrant. Add chopped kale and cook until wilted.
- Boil sweet potatoes until tender. Mash with a fork and season with salt and pepper.
- Serve grilled salmon with garlic kale and sweet potato mash.

Nutritional Info:

- Calories: 380 per serving
- Protein: 30g
- Carbohydrates: 30g
- Fat: 15g
- Fiber: 6g

6. Lentil Soup with Spinach and Turmeric

Ingredients:

- 1 cup lentils
- 4 cups vegetable broth
- 2 cups spinach
- 1 onion, diced
- 2 cloves garlic, minced
- 1 teaspoon turmeric powder
- Salt and pepper to taste

Preparation:

- In a pot, sauté diced onion and minced garlic until softened.
- Add lentils, vegetable broth, and turmeric powder. Bring to a boil, then simmer for 20-25 minutes until lentils are tender.
- Stir in spinach and cook until wilted.
- Season with salt and pepper before serving.

Nutritional Info:

- Calories: 250 per serving
- Protein: 18g
- Carbohydrates: 40g
- Fat: 1g
- Fiber: 16

7.   *Grilled Tofu Stir-Fry with Brown Rice*

Ingredients:

- 1 block tofu, pressed and cubed
- 2 cups mixed vegetables (broccoli, bell peppers, snap peas)
- 1 cup cooked brown rice
- 2 tablespoons low-sodium soy sauce
- 1 tablespoon sesame oil
- 2 cloves garlic, minced
- 1 teaspoon grated ginger
- Salt and pepper to taste

Preparation:

- Marinate tofu cubes in soy sauce, sesame oil, minced garlic, and grated ginger.
- Grill or pan-sear tofu until browned and crispy, about 5-7 minutes.
- Stir-fry mixed vegetables in a pan until tender-crisp.
- Serve grilled tofu and stir-fried vegetables over cooked brown rice.

Nutritional Info:

- Calories: 320 per serving
- Protein: 18g
- Carbohydrates: 45g
- Fat: 10g
- Fiber: 8g

8. Mediterranean Chickpea Salad

Ingredients:

- 2 cups cooked chickpeas
- 1 cup cherry tomatoes, halved
- 1 cucumber, diced
- 1/4 cup red onion, finely chopped
- 1/4 cup chopped fresh parsley
- 2 tablespoons olive oil
- 2 tablespoons lemon juice
- 1 teaspoon dried oregano
- Salt and pepper to taste

Preparation:

- Combine cooked chickpeas, cherry tomatoes, diced cucumber, chopped red onion, and chopped parsley in a large bowl.
- Drizzle olive oil and lemon juice over the salad. Sprinkle with dried oregano, salt, and pepper.
- Toss everything together until well combined.
- Serve as a refreshing salad for a light dinner option.

Nutritional Info:

- Calories: 280 per serving
- Protein: 12g
- Carbohydrates: 35g
- Fat: 12g
- Fiber: 10g

9. Baked Cod with Asparagus and Quinoa

Ingredients:

- 2 cod fillets
- 1 bunch asparagus, trimmed
- 1 cup quinoa
- 2 tablespoons lemon juice
- 2 tablespoons olive oil
- 2 cloves garlic, minced
- Salt and pepper to taste

Preparation:

- Preheat the oven to 400°F (200°C).
- Place cod fillets on a baking sheet. Drizzle with olive oil and lemon juice. Season with minced garlic, salt, and pepper.
- Arrange trimmed asparagus around the cod fillets on the baking sheet.
- Bake for 12-15 minutes until the cod is cooked through and flaky.
- Meanwhile, cook quinoa according to package instructions.
- Serve baked cod and asparagus over cooked quinoa.

Nutritional Info:

- Calories: 320 per serving
- Protein: 30g
- Carbohydrates: 30g
- Fat: 10g
- Fiber: 6g

10. Sweet Potato and Black Bean Tacos
Ingredients:

- 2 medium sweet potatoes, peeled and diced
- 1 tablespoon olive oil
- 1 teaspoon paprika
- 1 teaspoon cumin
- Salt and pepper to taste
- 1 can black beans, drained and rinsed
- 8 small corn tortillas
- 1/4 cup chopped cilantro
- 1 lime, cut into wedges

Preparation Method:

1. Preheat oven to 400°F (200°C).
2. Toss sweet potatoes with olive oil, paprika, cumin, salt, and pepper. Spread on a baking sheet and roast for 20 minutes.
3. Warm tortillas in a dry pan or microwave.
4. Fill tortillas with sweet potatoes and black beans. Top with cilantro and a squeeze of lime.

Cooking Time: 25 minutes

Nutritional Value: Per serving - Calories: 350, Protein: 10g, Fat: 9g, Carbohydrates: 60g

10 Delectable Anti-Inflammatory Snack Recipes

1. Turmeric Hummus

Ingredients:

- 1 can chickpeas, drained and rinsed
- 2 tablespoons tahini
- 2 tablespoons olive oil
- 1 lemon, juiced
- 1 teaspoon ground turmeric
- 1 clove garlic
- Salt to taste

Preparation Method:

1. Combine all ingredients in a food processor.
2. Blend until smooth, adding water as needed for desired consistency.

Cooking Time: 10 minutes

Nutritional Value: Per serving - Calories: 150, Protein: 4g, Fat: 8g, Carbohydrates: 14g

2. Avocado and Tomato Toast

Ingredients:

- 1 avocado, mashed

- 1 small tomato, sliced

- 2 slices whole grain bread

- Salt and pepper to taste

Preparation Method:

1. Toast the bread.

2. Spread mashed avocado on toast and top with tomato slices.

3. Season with salt and pepper.

Cooking Time: 5 minutes

Nutritional Value: Per serving - Calories: 200, Protein: 5g, Fat: 15g, Carbohydrates: 20g

3. Chia Seed Pudding

Ingredients:
- 1/4 cup chia seeds

- 1 cup almond milk

- 1 tablespoon honey

- 1/2 teaspoon vanilla extract

Preparation Method:

1. Mix all ingredients in a bowl.

2. Refrigerate for at least 4 hours or overnight.

Cooking Time: 5 minutes prep, 4 hours chill

Nutritional Value: Per serving - Calories: 180, Protein: 4g, Fat: 9g, Carbohydrates: 20g

4. Blueberry Almond Smoothie

Ingredients:
- 1 cup almond milk

- 1/2 cup blueberries
- 1 banana
- 1 tablespoon almond butter

Preparation Method:

1. Blend all ingredients until smooth.

Cooking Time: 5 minutes

Nutritional Value: Per serving - Calories: 250, Protein: 5g, Fat: 10g, Carbohydrates: 35g

5. Cucumber and Hummus Bites

Ingredients:
- 1 cucumber, sliced
- 1/2 cup hummus

Preparation Method:

1. Spread hummus on cucumber slices.

Cooking Time: 5 minutes

Nutritional Value: Per serving - Calories: 90, Protein: 3g, Fat: 4g, Carbohydrates: 12g

6. Walnut and Date Energy Balls

Ingredients:
- 1 cup walnuts
- 1 cup dates, pitted
- 1 tablespoon cocoa powder

Preparation Method:

1. Blend all ingredients in a food processor until sticky.
2. Roll into balls and refrigerate for 1 hour.

Cooking Time: 10 minutes prep, 1 hour chill

Nutritional Value: Per serving - Calories: 150, Protein: 3g, Fat: 10g, Carbohydrates: 20g

7. Apple Slices with Almond Butter

Ingredients:

- 1 apple, sliced
- 2 tablespoons almond butter

Preparation Method:

1. Spread almond butter on apple slices.

Cooking Time: 5 minutes

Nutritional Value: Per serving - Calories: 200, Protein: 4g, Fat: 10g, Carbohydrates: 30g

8. Roasted Chickpeas

Ingredients:

- 1 can chickpeas, drained and rinsed
- 1 tablespoon olive oil
- 1 teaspoon paprika
- 1/2 teaspoon cumin
- Salt to taste

Preparation Method:

1. Preheat oven to 400°F (200°C).
2. Toss chickpeas with olive oil and spices.
3. Spread on a baking sheet and roast for 20-30 minutes.

Cooking Time: 30 minutes

Nutritional Value: Per serving - Calories: 150, Protein: 6g, Fat: 6g, Carbohydrates: 20g

9. Berry Yogurt Parfait

Ingredients:

- 1 cup Greek yogurt

- 1/2 cup mixed berries

- 1 tablespoon honey

- 1/4 cup granola

Preparation Method:

1. Layer yogurt, berries, and granola in a glass.

2. Drizzle with honey.

Cooking Time: 5 minutes

Nutritional Value: Per serving - Calories: 250, Protein: 12g, Fat: 6g, Carbohydrates: 35g

10. Spiced Nuts

Ingredients:

- 2 cups mixed nuts

- 1 tablespoon olive oil

- 1 teaspoon paprika

- 1/2 teaspoon cayenne pepper

- Salt to taste

Preparation Method:

1. Preheat oven to 350°F (175°C).

2. Toss nuts with olive oil and spices.

3. Spread on a baking sheet and bake for 15 minutes.

Cooking Time: 15 minutes

Nutritional Value: Per serving - Calories: 200, Protein: 6g, Fat: 18g, Carbohydrates: 10g

10 Palatable Anti-Inflammatory Disease Dessert Recipes

1. Turmeric Golden Milk Ice Cream

Ingredients:

- 2 cups coconut milk
- 1/2 cup honey
- 1 teaspoon ground turmeric
- 1 teaspoon ground ginger
- 1/2 teaspoon cinnamon
- 1/4 teaspoon black pepper

Preparation Method:

1. Mix all ingredients in a saucepan and heat until combined.
2. Let the mixture cool, then churn in an ice cream maker according to the manufacturer's instructions.
3. Freeze until solid.

Preparation Time: 10 minutes prep, 4 hours chill

Nutritional Value: Per serving - Calories: 200, Protein: 1g, Fat: 14g, Carbohydrates: 22g

2. Blueberry Chia Pudding

Ingredients:

- 1/4 cup chia seeds
- 1 cup almond milk
- 1/2 cup blueberries
- 1 tablespoon honey

- 1/2 teaspoon vanilla extract

Preparation Method:

1. Mix all ingredients in a bowl.

2. Refrigerate for at least 4 hours or overnight.

Preparation Time: 5 minutes prep, 4 hours chill

Nutritional Value: Per serving - Calories: 180, Protein: 4g, Fat: 9g, Carbohydrates: 20g

3. Avocado Chocolate Mousse

Ingredients:

- 2 ripe avocados
- 1/4 cup cocoa powder
- 1/4 cup honey
- 1 teaspoon vanilla extract
- Pinch of salt

Preparation Method:

1. Blend all ingredients until smooth.

2. Refrigerate for 1 hour before serving.

Preparation Time: 10 minutes prep, 1 hour chill

Nutritional Value: Per serving - Calories: 220, Protein: 3g, Fat: 15g, Carbohydrates: 25g

4. Berry Coconut Popsicles

Ingredients:

- 1 cup mixed berries
- 1 cup coconut milk
- 2 tablespoons honey

Preparation Method:

1. Blend all ingredients until smooth.

2. Pour into popsicle molds and freeze for at least 4 hours.

Preparation Time: 10 minutes prep, 4 hours freeze

Nutritional Value: Per serving - Calories: 100, Protein: 1g, Fat: 7g, Carbohydrates: 10g

5. Oatmeal Banana Cookies

Ingredients:
- 2 ripe bananas
- 1 cup rolled oats
- 1/4 cup dark chocolate chips

Preparation Method:

1. Preheat oven to 350°F (175°C).

2. Mash bananas and mix with oats and chocolate chips.

3. Drop spoonfuls onto a baking sheet and bake for 15 minutes.

Preparation Time: 5 minutes prep, 15 minutes bake

Nutritional Value: Per serving - Calories: 90, Protein: 2g, Fat: 3g, Carbohydrates: 15g

6. Almond Butter Energy Balls

Ingredients:
- 1 cup rolled oats
- 1/2 cup almond butter
- 1/4 cup honey
- 1/4 cup dark chocolate chips

Preparation Method:

1. Mix all ingredients in a bowl.

2. Roll into balls and refrigerate for 1 hour.

Preparation Time: 10 minutes prep, 1 hour chill

Nutritional Value: Per serving - Calories: 150, Protein: 4g, Fat: 8g, Carbohydrates: 18g

7. Turmeric Ginger Smoothie

Ingredients:
- 1 cup almond milk
- 1 banana
- 1/2 teaspoon ground turmeric
- 1/2 teaspoon ground ginger
- 1 tablespoon honey

Preparation Method:
1. Blend all ingredients until smooth.

Preparation Time: 5 minutes

Nutritional Value: Per serving - Calories: 180, Protein: 2g, Fat: 4g, Carbohydrates: 35g

8. Coconut Mango Sorbet

Ingredients:
- 2 cups frozen mango chunks
- 1/2 cup coconut milk
- 1 tablespoon honey

Preparation Method:
1. Blend all ingredients until smooth.
2. Freeze for 1 hour before serving.

Preparation Time: 5 minutes prep, 1 hour freeze

Nutritional Value: Per serving - Calories: 120, Protein: 1g, Fat: 5g, Carbohydrates: 20g

9. Pumpkin Spice Chia Pudding

Ingredients:

- 1/4 cup chia seeds

- 1 cup almond milk

- 1/2 cup pumpkin puree

- 1 tablespoon honey

- 1/2 teaspoon cinnamon

Preparation Method:

1. Mix all ingredients in a bowl.

2. Refrigerate for at least 4 hours or overnight.

Preparation Time: 5 minutes prep, 4 hours chill

Nutritional Value: Per serving - Calories: 180, Protein: 4g, Fat: 8g, Carbohydrates: 24g

10. Dark Chocolate Avocado Truffles

Ingredients:

- 1 ripe avocado

- 1 cup dark chocolate, melted

- 1 teaspoon vanilla extract

- Cocoa powder for coating

Preparation Method:

1. Mash avocado and mix with melted chocolate and vanilla.

2. Refrigerate for 1 hour, then roll into balls and coat with cocoa powder.

Preparation Time: 10 minutes prep, 1 hour chill

Nutritional Value: Per serving - Calories: 120, Protein: 1g, Fat: 9g, Carbohydrates: 10g

Bonus 1: 6-Week Weekly Meal Planner

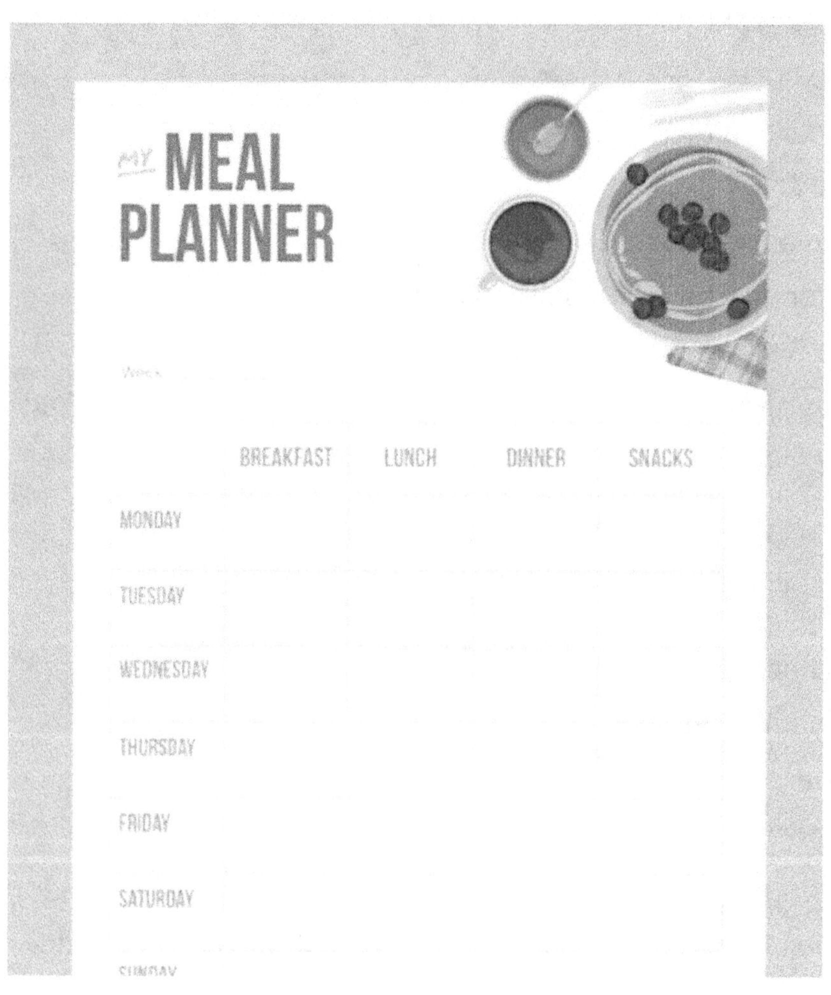

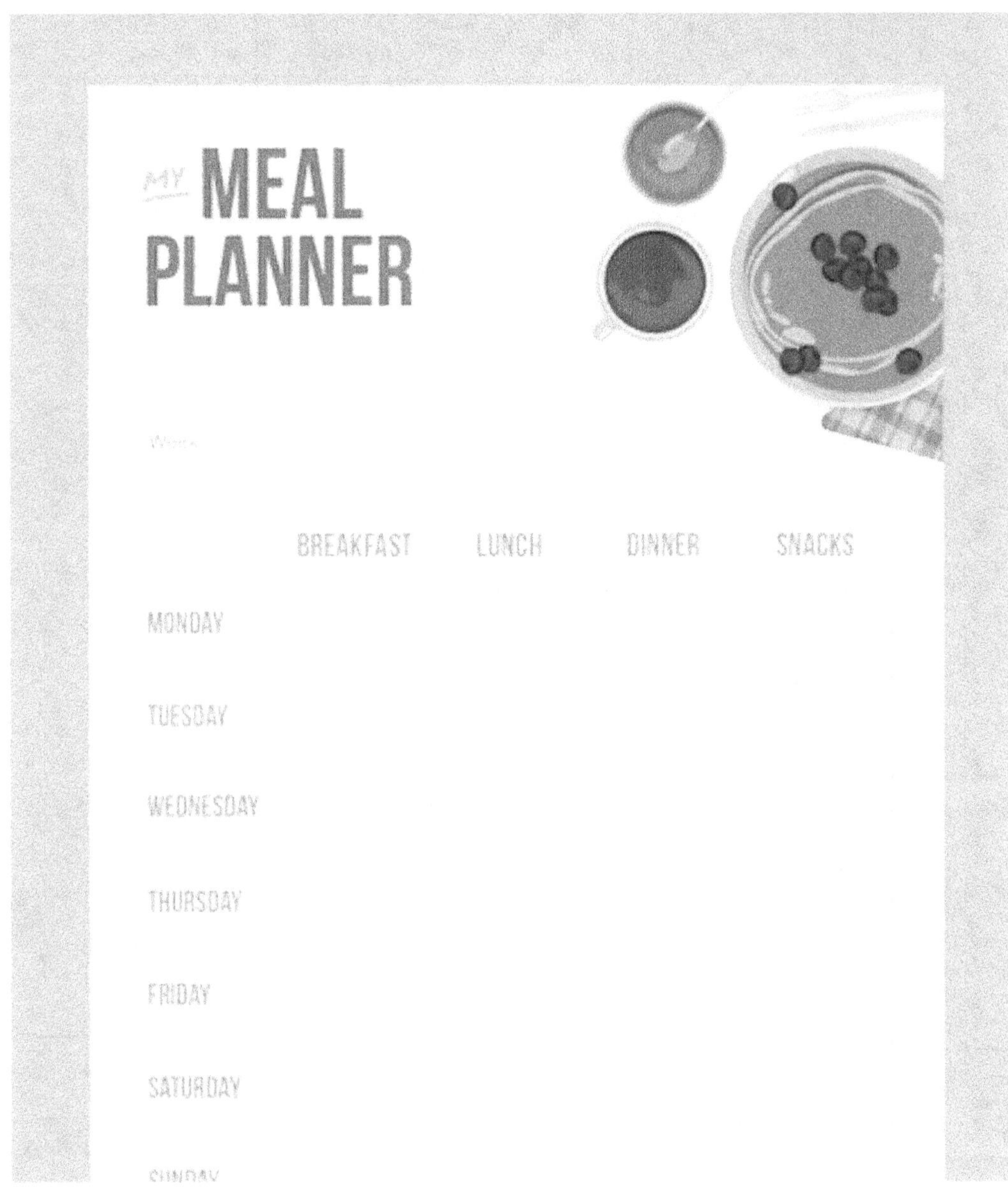
MY MEAL PLANNER

Week

BREAKFAST   LUNCH   DINNER   SNACKS

MONDAY

TUESDAY

WEDNESDAY

THURSDAY

FRIDAY

SATURDAY

SUNDAY

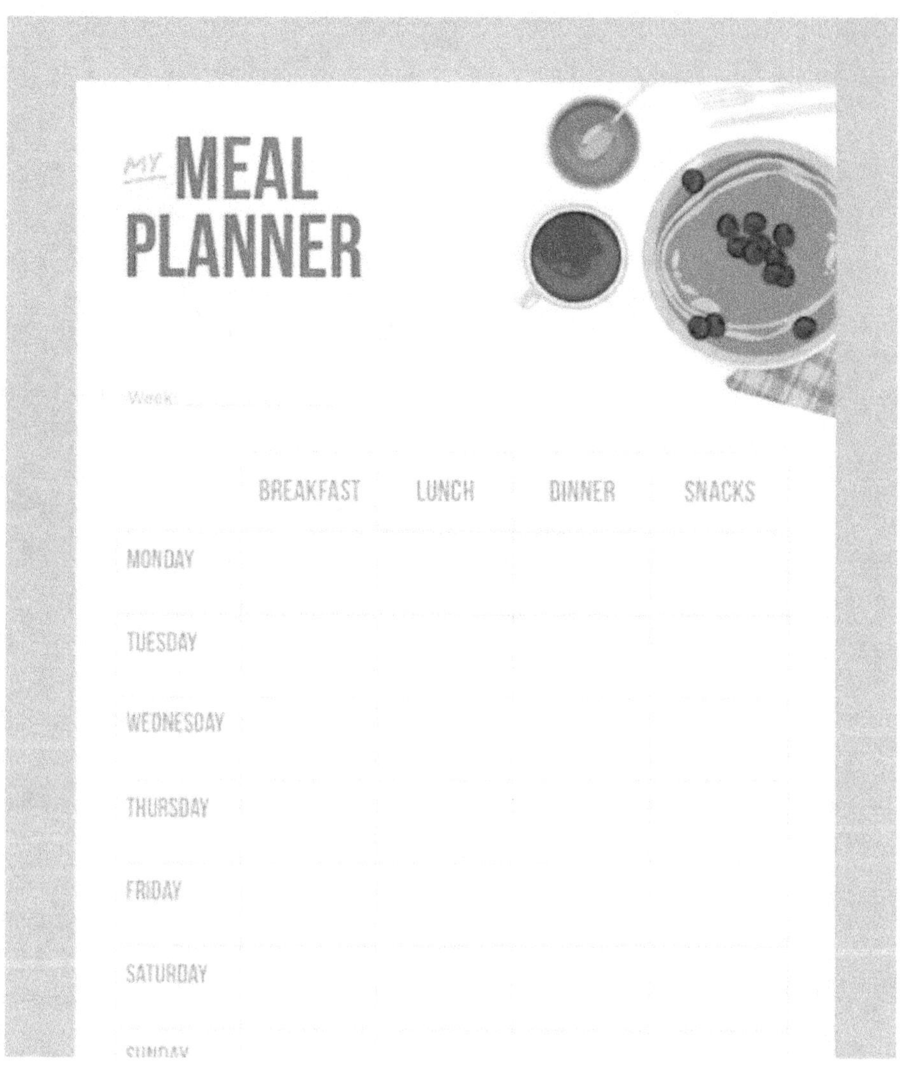
MY MEAL
PLANNER

Week:

BREAKFAST   LUNCH   DINNER   SNACKS

MONDAY

TUESDAY

WEDNESDAY

THURSDAY

FRIDAY

SATURDAY

SUNDAY

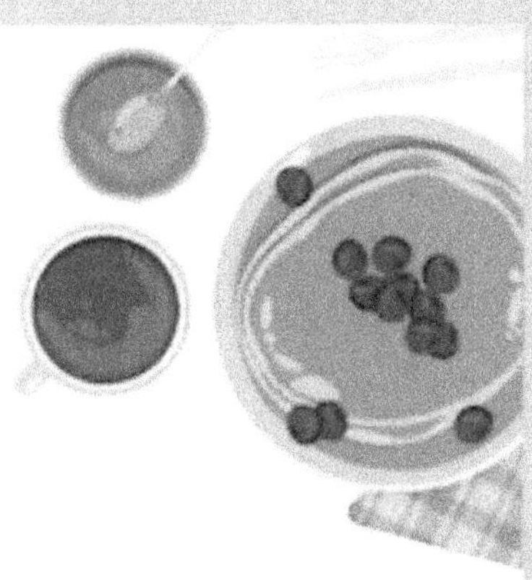

Week

	BREAKFAST	LUNCH	DINNER	SNACKS
MONDAY				
TUESDAY				
WEDNESDAY				
THURSDAY				
FRIDAY				
SATURDAY				
SUNDAY				

MY MEAL PLANNER

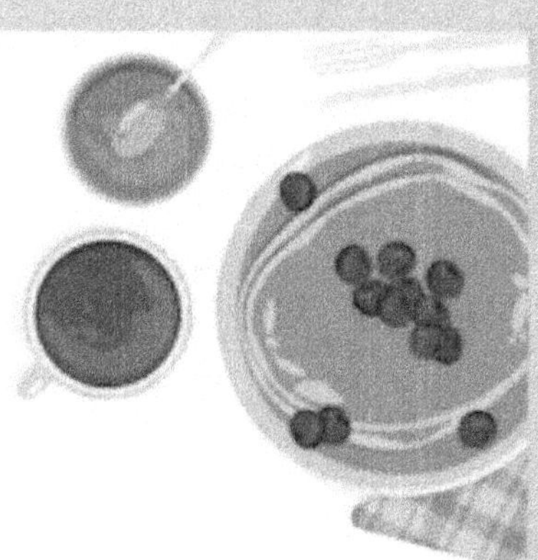

Week

	BREAKFAST	LUNCH	DINNER	SNACKS
MONDAY				
TUESDAY				
WEDNESDAY				
THURSDAY				
FRIDAY				
SATURDAY				
SUNDAY				

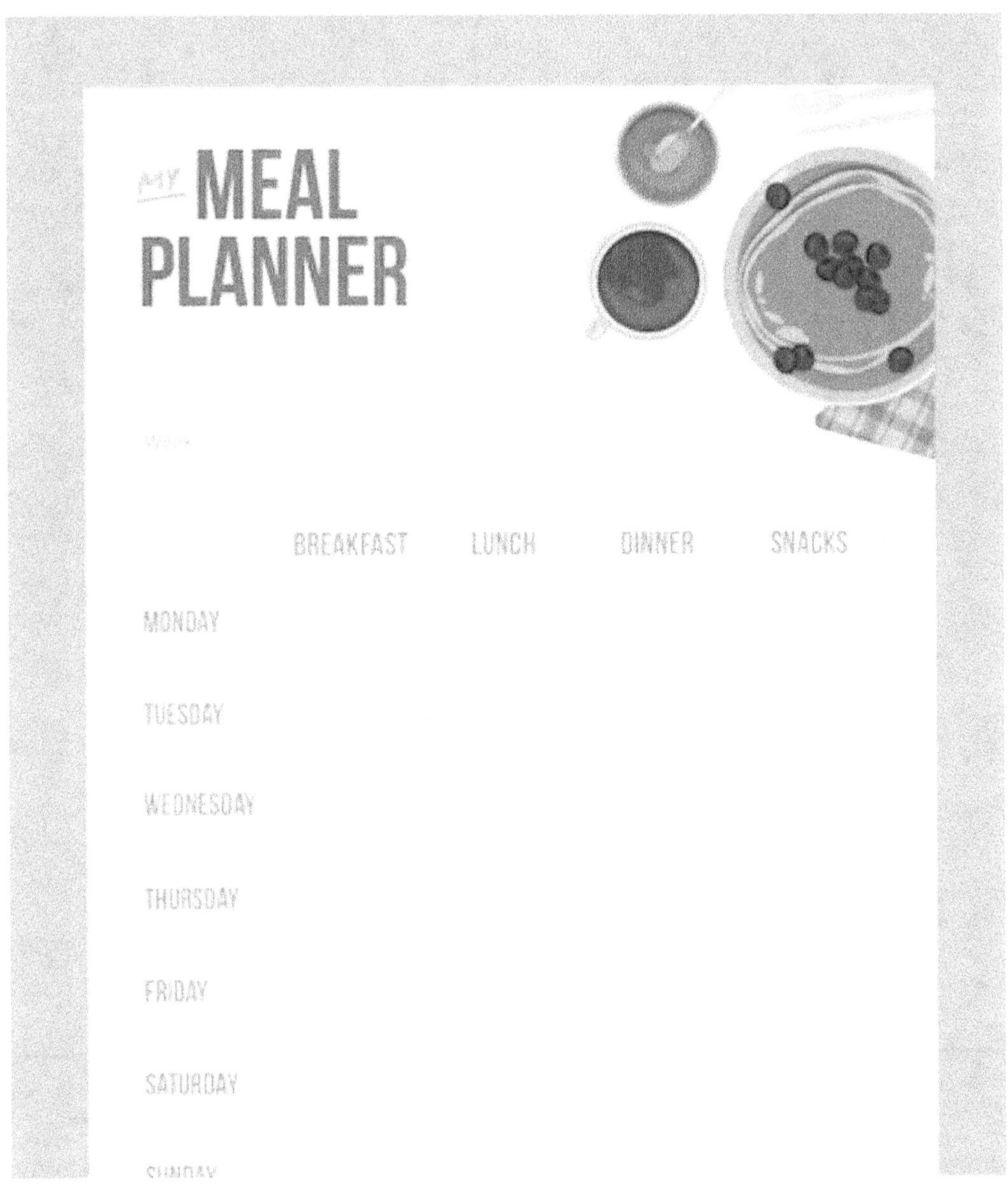

MY MEAL PLANNER

Week

BREAKFAST   LUNCH   DINNER   SNACKS

MONDAY

TUESDAY

WEDNESDAY

THURSDAY

FRIDAY

SATURDAY

SUNDAY

MY MEAL PLANNER

Week

	BREAKFAST	LUNCH	DINNER	SNACKS
MONDAY				
TUESDAY				
WEDNESDAY				
THURSDAY				
FRIDAY				
SATURDAY				
SUNDAY				

Bonus 2: 6-Week Meal Monitoring Schedule

WEEKLY SCHEDULE

TIME	MONDAY	TUESDAY	WEDNESDAY	THURSDAY	FRIDAY	SATURDAY	SUNDAY
7 AM							
8 AM							
9 AM							
10 AM							
11 AM							
12 PM							
1 PM							
2 PM							
3 PM							
4 PM							
5 PM							
6 PM							
7 PM							
8 PM							
9 PM							
10 PM							

WEEKLY SCHEDULE

TIME	MONDAY	TUESDAY	WEDNESDAY	THURSDAY	FRIDAY	SATURDAY	SUNDAY
7 AM							
8 AM							
9 AM							
10 AM							
11 AM							
12 PM							
1 PM							
2 PM							
3 PM							
4 PM							
5 PM							
6 PM							
7 PM							
8 PM							
9 PM							
10 PM							

WEEKLY SCHEDULE

TIME	MONDAY	TUESDAY	WEDNESDAY	THURSDAY	FRIDAY	SATURDAY	SUNDAY
7 AM							
8 AM							
9 AM							
10 AM							
11 AM							
12 PM							
1 PM							
2 PM							
3 PM							
4 PM							
5 PM							
6 PM							
7 PM							
8 PM							
9 PM							
10 PM							

WEEKLY SCHEDULE

TIME	MONDAY	TUESDAY	WEDNESDAY	THURSDAY	FRIDAY	SATURDAY	SUNDAY
7 AM							
8 AM							
9 AM							
10 AM							
11 AM							
12 PM							
1 PM							
2 PM							
3 PM							
4 PM							
5 PM							
6 PM							
7 PM							
8 PM							
9 PM							
10 PM							

WEEKLY SCHEDULE

TIME	MONDAY	TUESDAY	WEDNESDAY	THURSDAY	FRIDAY	SATURDAY	SUNDAY
7 AM							
8 AM							
9 AM							
10 AM							
11 AM							
12 PM							
1 PM							
2 PM							
3 PM							
4 PM							
5 PM							
6 PM							
7 PM							
8 PM							
9 PM							
10 PM							

WEEKLY SCHEDULE

TIME	MONDAY	TUESDAY	WEDNESDAY	THURSDAY	FRIDAY	SATURDAY	SUNDAY
7 AM							
8 AM							
9 AM							
10 AM							
11 AM							
12 PM							
1 PM							
2 PM							
3 PM							
4 PM							
5 PM							
6 PM							
7 PM							
8 PM							
9 PM							
10 PM							

NOTE TO THE READER

Dear Reader,

Thank you for choosing my book to read.

As a nutritionist author, reviews are helpful to me. If you derived value from this book, I would be so grateful if you would leave a review on Amazon.com.

If you are experiencing acid reflux or GERD/LPR and other related diseases associated with aging and would need help to manage or reverse this condition by following a tested and proven dietary guideline, I recommend this helpful book in my library titled: "Acid Reflux Reversal Manual and Cookbook". This comprehensive guide offers not only relief but a long-term solution to your acid reflux woes. To have access to this book, please click here.

I love to hear any feedback about any of my books and enjoy interacting with my readers. So please feel free to e-mail me at mary.d.johnson@gmail.com.

Thanks a million!

Mary D. Johnson

CONCLUSION

Congratulations on reaching the end of this book, "The Ultimate Anti-inflammatory Diet Cookbook for Seniors"! You now possess the knowledge and tools to transform your health through delicious, nutrient-packed recipes designed to combat inflammation. By incorporating these meals into your daily routine, you can reduce pain, boost your energy, and reclaim the vibrant life you deserve.

Remember, the journey to better health is a marathon, not a sprint. Embrace these recipes as part of a holistic lifestyle change that includes regular exercise, adequate sleep, and stress management. Share these meals with loved ones and inspire others to join you on this path to wellness.

As you continue exploring and experimenting in the kitchen, let the flavors and benefits of anti-inflammatory foods be your guide. Stay curious, stay motivated, and most importantly, stay committed to your health.

Thank you for choosing this cookbook as your companion on this journey. Here's to a healthier, happier, and more vibrant you! Don't forget to revisit these pages for inspiration and to remind yourself of the positive changes you've made. Happy cooking and good health!

www.ingramcontent.com/pod-product-compliance
Lightning Source LLC
Chambersburg PA
CBHW081226260726
48653CB00010BB/3814